FIRE-UP YOUR FAT BURN!
Super-Easy Quick Tips, Strategies and Goals for Fast Weight Loss

By Lori Shemek, PhD, CNC

As the Fitness Expert for *Lifetime TV's "The Balancing Act"* I think Dr. Lori's book is a must buy for anyone who needs a quick guide on how to get on track and start seeing the results you want...quickly! ~Troy J. Hines, LIFETIME TV Fitness Trainer

"This publication has been the most effective and results driven weight loss program I have ever tried! After gaining some unwanted pounds and trying all the no-carb, high protein, WW, paleo and other programs, Dr. Lori's is the best! I've lost 40 lbs!" ~Andrea Feldman

"Power-packed book on getting fat off your body fast!, Dr. Lori's excellent book, Fire-Up Your Fat Burn!, is a wealth of information on how anyone can increase their metabolic rate fast and the right way! That includes building muscle so that sustained fat loss can occur. ~Robert Choat, America's #1 Mind-Body Transformation Expert, author of 'Mind Your Own Fitness.

"This book is just what you need if you want to be fit and not fat. .. I started reading this book last weekend and I have not been able to stop. This book is a must read!" ~Irvin Eatman, former NFL Player and Coach

"This book is quick, POWERFUL and straight to the gut! This is not a book filled with a bunch of fluff and hype. I have lost 30 pounds without going on a diet or making radical changes to my life style with this book. I love the book and the advice provided because it works!" ~Scott Whitelaw author of "Earl's Pearls, Jewels of Wisdom Worth Passing On"

"I've been reading Dr. Lori's book and can honestly say that I've never felt better in my life. I've lost 40 plus pounds, I eat three meals a day, I am never hungry, nor do I ever feel deprived. The weight and inches are falling off! If it worked for me, it will work for you too!!! Just try it!" ~Kathy Sistilli

"Quick, easy read! You'll want to start your changes today! And no need to get out your calculator...you won't be counting calories. . SIMPLE changes, BIG results! Oh, but it does have some side effects - losing weight and feeling great!" ~Angie F.

"This book is chock full of information. It is a very easy, straight forward read. Each chapter has tons of information that is easy to understand and easy to implement in your life. The author takes you through what to eat (and why), what types of exercises to do, and what types of supplements benefit your health " ~Glenneth Reed

"I just read this book last night and It is broken down to exactly what you need to do. This will change your entire outlook on fitness and nutrition. This book illustrates is the plan to put you onto that road, and quickly. A must read for beginners and experts alike. This author definitely knows her information and has done her research in all areas of fitness and nutrition" ~Doug Oz

"Lori's Advice is timeless, easy and AWESOME! "Fire-Up Your Fat Burn!" is the ultimate guide to losing weight and keeping it off. I came to Lori after battling cancer and I wouldn't be where I am today without Lori. I can't recommend this book enough" ~Laurie Lieker

"A practical guide to raising metabolism and burning fat. This book from Dr. Lori Shemek tells you exactly what you need to know to create a life of optimal health, it an essential and practical guide to raising your metabolism and burning fat. Not only do I highly recommend you read this book I suggest you use it as a reference to help you reach your goals." ~Jason Owen

" A Great book, very informative. Once I read it I was revved up and ready to try to lose weight again! Easy to follow the daily meal plans - can't wait to see the results!" ~Val

"Helpful and easy to follow! Enjoyed this book! It's a quick read and provided a lot of helpful information in easy-to-follow lists. Makes it seem easy!" ~Shawna Hansen

" I've read numerous books on the subject in order to be aware of resources to refer to clients and for my own personal weight management goals! I can think of no other book on the subject that is as user-friendly as Fire Up Your Fat Burn! Lori has knocked a home run with this book! " ~Mark Hundley, Author of 'Awaken To Good Mourning'

"Amazing! A must have book! This book ROCKS! I love that Lori is right to the point. It's an easy read and you don't have to read 400 pages to get all the information you need. The menu's, grocery list and training tips are great!" ~Kelly Leustek

"Great Resource!" This book is the best source of inspiration and information! After losing 40lbs, I had hit that plateau that we've all heard about and probably met before. No matter what I tried, nothing worked. Then I found "Fire Up Your Fat Burn"and what profound difference that made. I've gotten past that plateau and lost an additional 10lbs! I've never read any other publication that went into such great detail as "Fat Burn!" has" ~Rob Byrd

This book is quite practical for those of us who not only want to sheds some extra pounds but eat healthy as well. It is a very clear, concise approach to good nutrition The regimen and menu recommendations are *very* doable with not too many restrictions. highly recommend this book...Enjoy!" ~Jim Faas

.
"A straightforward guide to living a healthy life. A diet as a way of life rather than deprivation. I appreciate the explanations of "why" that are included in each chapter. I have read articles by Dr. Lori Shemek so didn't hesitate to download this book. Reading it for the second time to make sure I didn't miss anything!" ~Suzanne

"My fat burn is on fire! There are so many "thick" books out there with "thick" prices on them. A bunch of useless filler pages with little content. Dr. Shemek hits it on the head, the first time! Her book is an easy read with many useful tips. I have changed up my training program and incorporated her suggestions for a leaner body. GREAT book, and I highly recommend it!" ~Mark K. Rickert

Published in the United States

First Publishing Date: August, 2012

ISBN-13: 978-1479170289

ISBN-10: 1479170283

Disclaimer

All material provided is for informational and educational purposes only, and in no way is any of the content to be construed as medical advice or instruction. These statements and the supplements mentioned within are not intended to diagnose, treat, cure or prevent any disease and no action should be taken solely on the contents of this publication. Consult your physician or a qualified health professional on any matters regarding your health and wellbeing. Lori Shemek, PhD does not assume any liability for the information contained herein, be it direct, indirect, consequential, special, exemplary or other damages.

Developments in medical research may impact the health and nutritional advice that appears here. No assurance can be given that the advice contained in this site will always include the most recent findings or developments with respect to the particular material.

If you think you may have a medical emergency, call your doctor or 911 immediately. Lori Shemek, PhD is not a licensed medical, health professional. Her doctorate is in counseling psychology. Reliance on any information provided by Lori Shemek, PhD is solely at your own risk.

Forward

Having seen Dr. Lori Shemek in action as she helps so many people in losing weight in a healthy manner is amazing. This book is a taste of some of her insider knowledge on what it takes to burn fat fast. There's been a lot of misconception as to what it takes to burn off fat and look great. Dr. Shemek has been able to distill it down to its essence so that anyone wanting to "burn it off", can.

You can either go on so-called "yo-yo diets" or outdated USDA guidelines. Dr. Shemek continues her search into the latest research on getting healthy and fit. It's time you benefit from her hard and dedicated work.

In today's fast-paced world, it's wonderful that she's been able to come up with this solution that will help many. Those of you that have kept up with the latest news regarding obesity will know that the latest predictions that in the United States, 42% of Americans will be obese by 2030. Dr. Shemek has made it part of her mission to help educate her clients and the population to lose the weight and get fit.

I highly recommend this book as a resource to those that are looking to living a lifestyle that is healthy and fit. Just do it!

Bob Choat
Mind-Body Transformation Expert

Introduction

If you are reading this book, then chances are you are ready to melt the fat, trim up and finally change your body. You have probably experienced your share of diets, quick weight loss plans, and programs that take the fun out of eating - not to mention the dollars spent..and you are sick of it! I don't blame you. I have listened to my clients' stories and I have witnessed the devastation, emotionally and physically, that results from too much dieting, choosing quick diet programs, fad diets and more.

This book is not a diet nor is it a waste of time. What you are holding in your hand is your new life, a life that holds a slimmer and healthier you.

The information contained within this book is a collection of years of research and client experience to help you create successful, lasting fat loss.

FIRE-UP YOUR FAT BURN! is the latest information to date on fat loss in the form of super-easy quick tips, strategies and goals.

You are going to get from me, all the tips and insight you need to lose weight. I've covered food, exercise, your mind-set, and more. You now hold the key to successful fat loss. I'm confident you have all the information necessary to make changes that will fire-up your fat burn and lead to the changes you need to live our best life.

Here's to your best health,
Lori Shemek, Ph.D., CNC

Table of Contents

"There are only two options regarding commitment; you're either in or you're out. There's no such thing as life in-between."
~Pat Riley

Congratulations! You have taken a huge step by joining many others who are now enjoying and experiencing weight loss and optimal health. What you are holding in your hand, FIRE-UP YOUR FAT BURN! Contains everything you need: the tools, content and accountability that will take you right to your desired goal - easily and quickly. Okay, let's get started!

In life, there are two things you can control:

- How much you move your body

- What and how much food you eat

Ask yourself, if you continue what you are doing and continue eating what you are eating, will you look and feel any different five years down the road? Now, I want you to really focus on this here. Envision yourself fatter, less energetic, and struggling with everyday tasks, foggy thinking and just plain miserable - a poorer quality of life. Understand that this is a real possible scenario if you continue to make the same lifestyle choices - would you want your child to take that path in life? You must value yourself enough to realize that you are worthy of optimal health and weight loss - you deserve it. You don't deserve to be fat or burdened with ill health. If you don't take care of your health..who will?

A healthy lifestyle, full of energy and vitality, takes focus and follow through initially. But, you know what? You can do this!! After approximately 3 weeks, you will have integrated new habits in your life that will not only create weight loss now, but create optimal health as well, that will serve you for the rest of your life. Every single change you make..starting right now..will take you to fat burn success! There is no reason for you to count calories - STOP COUNTING CALORIES! (Who wants to do that??) or resort to unhealthy diets - fads and otherwise.

The main reason people are overweight? It's not what you think. It's not about the calories, it's not about overeating and it's not about the exercise - It is about the foods you are eating that are the main cause of your weight gain. Now, there are other factors that play into this as well, but it really is about how the foods you eat, how even so-called 'healthy foods' affect your weight. Eating the right way will help you burn fat immediately and easily.

One important key to creating success with your weight loss goals is through accountability. The use of this book and other tools available (see Appendix A), such as the included **Nutrition Fast Trac™** , you are engaging the very important key of accountability.

Another important key in creating a successful

outcome with your fat loss goal is: consistency. This means tracking your nutrition progress through the Nutrition Fast Trac™ on a daily basis or with others like it listed on the resources page of this book. Consistency in action and consistency in tracking will carry you straight to fat burn success. Every step you take in that direction, whether big or small, is one step closer to your goal.

Quick Success Strategies

- **Reduce Cellular inflammation.** *Your #1 key to weight loss success is to reduce inflammation in your body.* Inflammation is the core cause of weight gain. Fat creates inflammation and inflammation creates fat - a vicious cycle that can be broken. Fat cells produce inflammatory molecules that trigger inflammation in the body, slow the metabolism and thus, contribute to weight gain. The tips, strategies and goals you find here will help you to reverse and prevent the inflammation that is responsible for your weight gain.

- **Utilize Accountability.** Each week choose just one new *"Healthy Focus"* to integrate every day via the **Nutrition Fast Trac**™ . This doesn't mean to disregard the other important healthful choices - it is simply a success strategy to integrate important weight loss choices slowly (key) to ensure they become an established part of your life. These *"Healthy Focus"* choices will become automatic if you are consistent.

  - **Eating five times a day:** Breakfast, Snack, Lunch, Snack, and Dinner are critical in promoting weight loss. With each meal and snack it is important to consume a lean protein, a complex carbohydrate and a healthy fat.

You must consume them every 3 hours. Eating five times a day and adding protein to each meal will stabilize your blood sugar - *stable blood sugar is key to promoting weight loss*. Stable blood sugar inhibits inflammation and **cellular inflammation is the core cause of most weight gain, illness, disease and faster aging.** By feeding your body throughout the day, you will not be as hungry and vulnerable to making poor food choices and you will keep your metabolism humming.

- **Portion Control:** Portion Control is key to creating weight loss. You want to see those abs don't you? A clenched fist is roughly the portion size for a serving of carbohydrates and the palm of your hand and thickness is roughly the portion size of your lean protein. (See Resource page).

- **The "Plate Method"** A simple and highly effective guide for portion control for weight loss is the **"Plate Method"** Make certain that half your plate is veggies, 1/4 complex carbohydrates such as brown rice or whole wheat and 1/4 lean protein.

- **Consume healthy fat daily** - examples: avocado, nuts or seeds, cold water fish, olive oil, flaxseed oil, natural peanut butter (no sugar in the peanut butter) or fish oil supplements.

- **Drink Water:** Drink a minimum of half your body weight in water ounces. For example, if you weigh 120 lbs. you will drink a minimum of 60 ounces each day to boost your metabolism. Now, I know this may seem like a lot of water, but starting off slowly..will get you there successfully and you'll be a water rock star melting the fat off!

- **Eat Protein With Every Meal**. The math is simple: eating protein stimulates Glucagon release = fat release. Fat release is a good thing. Protein also reduces the insulin response - important because insulin is your fat storage hormone.

- **Avoid** refined carbohydrates such as white sugar, white rice, white flour products, and processed foods. Note that I'm not saying to minimize your intake of these 'foods,' I'm saying to avoid them...run the other way when you see them.

- **Move Your Body**. Exercise stimulates glucagon release which burns fat and sugar. Incorporate the quickest, most effective fat burning exercise: Interval Training.

Eat Like a Champion

Olympic Swimmer, Dara Torres, continued to compete at world class levels well into her 40's. In 2008, she became the oldest female Olympic swimmer in history at the age of 41. Perhaps what will always be remembered about her is how she trained. Despite being a mother and other things in her life, Dara trains at a high level (as of this writing).

Having first competed in the Olympics in 1984, she went made the decision to compete in the 2008 and 2012 Games. In 2008, she won 2 silver medals. Now, in 2012, she is in a fight to make the team as she is feeling her age. Hers is a story of inspiration for those that are older. It takes dedication and perseverance to do what she does and this is where nutrition really counts.

Olympic level athletes have a baseline diet where they start from and it's not much different than what the average person should be eating. Dara Torres once said that diets are important for health and fitness. And during an interview in 2010 she said, "I spend part of each day working out in the pool, which is a great way to stay healthy. I also make sure to eat plenty of protein and vegetables, stretch after I swim, give my body plenty of time to recover -- and spend plenty of time with my daughter, which always makes me smile and relaxes me!"

"With the epidemic of childhood obesity and the increasing body-fat percentage of all Americans, obesity is definitely one of the biggest healthcare concerns facing Americans today." -Dara Torres

So it is the same for all of us. Now it is time for you to eat like a champion. Let's get you started today.

Breakfast

It is very important that you eat breakfast every day. Okay, you may not be used to eating breakfast. But just look to people who have achieved their weight loss goals - chances are they eat breakfast. Research shows the people who are most successful with their weight loss and fitness eat breakfast. The reason for this is that you are stabilizing your blood sugar. *Even if you do not feel hungry*, your blood sugar is low because you have been 8 hours without nourishment. This will lead, later in the day, to poor food choices (Remember Inflammation? Junk food is inflammation's best friend).

Always pair a complex carbohydrate (sprouted whole grain product, whole grains, fruit, veggies, beans) with a protein for optimal satiation and to stabilize your blood sugar.

Breakfast Examples:

- One half of a sprouted whole wheat English muffin or whole wheat bread with 2 tablespoons of natural peanut butter (**NO** sugar or added fat in peanut butter).

- A scramble wrap: a whole wheat low-carb tortilla filled with 1 whole egg and 1 egg white scrambled, a slice of avocado and a strip of turkey bacon.

- A filling toasted egg and cheese sandwich: 2 slices of whole grain thin bread, 1 egg and 1 slice of low fat cheese or low fat shredded cheese. *Thin bread brands are available at most grocery stores in the bread section.

Protein is critical in helping to melt the fat. **By adding protein you will be putting the brakes on your craving for carbohydrates.**

Breakfast protein can include: whey protein or any type of protein powder. Just mix it with low fat (no sugar) almond milk, skim milk or water. Whey is *extremely* beneficial for boosting your metabolism, building muscle, improving digestion and immunity. The more muscle you have the more calories you burn - muscle burns calories even at rest. You can use the whey protein for breakfast, lunch or dinner. Eggs, cottage cheese, Low-fat cheese, yogurt, vegetarian protein sources (beans, nuts, seeds, soy bacon, tempeh, quinoa etc.), are other excellent sources.

Lunch

Lunch Examples:

- A turkey sandwich with lean turkey on two thin slices of sprouted whole wheat bread is an excellent choice to help you feel full. Add a couple slices of avocado for your beneficial fat and even more fiber. To round out this healthful meal, add veggies in any form. You can also drink your veggies too! Choose either fresh veggie juice, low-sodium V8 or low-sodium tomato juice. Phytonutrients in veggies and veggie juices also help with weight loss and lowering inflammation via their ability to protect and reverse the oxidant onslaught to our cells.

- Try leftover healthy soups or stews from the night before. Again, if protein seems to be lacking, please use protein in powder form which is easily assimilated by the body.

- Take a very hollowed out high fiber roll and fill it 4 slices of turkey, guacamole and melt 1 slice of low fat jack cheese on top. Pair your roll with V8 juice or a piece of whole fruit.

- Try a large salad filled with leafy greens and topped with chopped-up vegetables and add lean chicken, or a handful of beans for protein. For salad dressing, avoid fatty dressings such as white dressings. Use a teaspoon of olive oil/flax oil and lemon or lime juice.

- Frozen entrees, such as Lean Cuisine or Healthy Choice are fine in a pinch, (they also teach portion control) just pair it with a veggie (a salad, carrot and celery sticks, etc.) or a veggie drink such as low-sodium V-8 juice. Whole fruit is another excellent choice.

If pairing fruit with a meal such as your lunch, choose lower sugar fruits such as berries, whole apple, orange, or pears. Higher sugar fruits such as bananas, cantaloupe, watermelon, pineapple are allowing a higher sugar intake and sugar equals inflammation. Have a small portion of these fruits only occasionally.

With each meal it is important to add veggies to your dish - an easy way to get your veggies in each day. Veggies are complex carbohydrates, which means they slow down the release of sugar in your body - **a fast release of sugar is what makes us fat**. As I have mentioned - it is vital that you get more protein and healthy fat to help satiate you as well prevent excess intake of carbohydrates. Too many carbohydrates will raise your blood sugar (protein does not do this) and this creates a steep drop in blood sugar - this action of spiking blood sugar and the inevitable precipitous drop is inflammation and inflammation is responsible for your weight gain (along with a whole host of other illness or diseases).

Dinner

Dinner Examples:

- A quick chicken sauté with olive oil, summer squash, black olives, onions, spices and lean skinless, boneless chicken breast poured over 1/2 cup of brown rice or pasta.

- Marinara sauce, shrimp, olive oil and 1/2 cup sprouted whole wheat pasta and salad.

- Turkey burger made with lean ground turkey breast, two slices of avocado on high fiber very hollowed-out whole grain bun, V-8 juice, and you have a healthful meal.

Remember, be creative! Yes you are creative! You can switch up breakfast for dinner, dinner for lunch, lunch for breakfast etc. You do not have to eat traditional foods for each meal. Take the time to easily and quickly create healthy soups and stews, made in advance, that you can freeze in individual zip locks and heat up quickly. Add a serving of fat-melting brown rice (NOT white rice - NO) for a complex carb/fiber a veggie of your choice and you have a healthful complete meal that will promote fat-burning success!!

When dining out, always search for the non-fried foods such as baked, steamed, or grilled. Remember to also look to 'sides' to fulfill your veggie, protein, and complex carbohydrate requirements. Avoid the bread or tortilla chips if offered. In these instances, **Be Strong**. What do you want your body, your health, your life to look like 5 years down the road? Focus on this and feel the emotion behind your visualization.

Snacks:

Snacks are important for successful weight loss! Snacking will help keep you on track by preventing dips in your blood sugar that lead to fatigue and cravings. Snacking will also prevent you from becoming so overly hungry that you overeat and make poor food choices.

I've seen how easily a bag of Fritos can disappear. Mindless eating is often the downfall of successful weight loss. Now I know you have good intentions...but we know all too well about good intentions. You may start out saying you are going to eat only a few of your favorite crackers, only to finish the entire box without even thinking about it. Obviously, this example isn't the healthy snacking that can help you reach your fitness or weight loss goals.

It is important to snack! Be mindful of snacking between meals. You should have 2 snacks a day. This will not only keep you from overeating, but prevent you from making poor food choices by balancing your blood sugar. Snacking will boost your metabolism and fire-up that fat burn!

Remove sugar and snacks with sugar from your diet. Whole fruit is a better choice however and I recommend you include it as a snack each day.

Do not drink fruit juice - it is metabolized quickly - just like sugar. Yes, it contains vitamins and minerals, but it is just a step up from a coke. So **avoid** fruit juice! Remember: the way sugar and juice are metabolized creates inflammation in the body and an excess of insulin. This means weight gain.

For weight loss success, always pair a protein choice along with a carbohydrate with every snack and meal.

Repeat: Snacks stabilize the blood sugar which is the root of overeating and making poor food choices = weight gain. Not only does snacking stabilize blood sugar - it boosts your metabolism as well!

Snack Examples:

- A half of a sprouted whole wheat English muffin topped with a slice of tomato and 2 oz. of turkey

- 1 tablespoon of peanut butter to one serving of whole grain crackers.

- A half-cup serving of low-fat cottage cheese mixed with one quarter cup of fresh blueberries or raspberries

- A packet of plain quick-cooking steel-cut oatmeal cooked with one-half of a cup of skim or no sugar almond milk.

- Whole grain crackers topped with low-fat cheese or peanut butter

- An apple and one string cheese

- A low-carb tortilla rolled with a lean lunch meat.

- A small handful of nuts and raspberries.

- Hummus with 10 baby carrots and a whole red pepper cut into strips

- Two cups of air-popped popcorn mixed with 2 tbsp. of grated Parmesan cheese.

YOUR FAT LOSS FOUNDATION

Fruits and Vegetables

It is important to incorporate a minimum of 2 1/2 cups of vegetables each day. One serving = 1/2 cup.

Vegetables are full of antioxidants, vitamins, minerals and fiber that will take you to fat loss success. Without an abundance of these nutrients, we are at risk not only for *weight gain*...but serious diseases such as obesity, cardiovascular disease, cancer, diabetes, Alzheimer's disease, hypertension, cataracts, faster aging and more.

Your ability to stay ***free of weight gain*** and these diseases depends upon an adequate intake of protective antioxidants (chemicals capable of disarming free-radicals) to prevent the free-radicals from damaging your body and causing inflammation. Free-radicals are the body's equivalent to nuclear waste and this means you will pack on the pounds.

There are many ways to incorporate fruits and vegetables into your diet. The best way to ensure your optimum intake is to add them to every meal. They can be added to sandwiches, soups and stews, roasted or steamed etc. Carrots, for example, can be shredded and added to a myriad of dishes including: Chili, soups, or stuffed into a whole wheat wrap. A mixture of vegetables can be diced and added to scrambled eggs or an omelet. 8 ounces of vegetable juice is considered a serving of vegetables and extremely healthful.

If you do not like veggies or not used to eating them, slowly integrate veggies into your diet. It may take a little while for you to acclimate to the taste and consistent use of veggies, but doing so will result in weight loss with consistent use.

Protein

A serving of protein is 3 - 4 ounces or the size and thickness of your palm (see resource section for guide).

It is important that you have protein with every meal and snack. Protein is an important part of a healthy diet and key in weight loss assuming the carbohydrate intake is not in excess.

Protein stimulates the release of glucagon, which stimulates the liver to release stored carbohydrates. Glucagon also inhibits the release of insulin. By controlling your intake of protein and spreading it throughout the day, you can constantly produce adequate amounts of glucagon.

Unlike high carbohydrate diets, protein triggers a response that stimulates the release of glucagon, **a hormone that helps us to burn previously stored fat**.

Ensure that your protein choice is a low-fat lean source such as: skinless chicken, turkey breast (skinless, roasted), all lean meats (90% lean), lean lunch meats, low-fat cottage cheese, low-fat cheeses, whey protein powder and even peanut butter despite its high fat content and nuts or seeds (healthy fat helps you feel fuller thereby tamping down your desire for food) - these will all help you reduce your weight. Remember to minimize your high fat dairy intake - opt for low-fat instead.

Do you know that there is more calcium in fruits and vegetables than milk or milk products?

*Protein bars and drinks typically have a lot of sugar. Make sure there is no listed sugar when looking at the nutrition label.

Complex Carbohydrates

A serving of complex carbohydrates = 1/2 cup.

A major key in successful weight loss is fiber. Fiber creates fullness and stabilizes your blood sugar. Complex carbohydrates do just that because they are high in fiber and are also very important to optimal health.

Examples of complex carbohydrates are: beans - all beans (black beans, lima beans, white beans, red beans etc), all *whole* sprouted grains (*whole* sprouted wheat products, oats, brown rice, quinoa, spelt, rye and more), legumes (split peas, lentils etc.) and all fruits and vegetables.

Complex carbohydrates are "slow-releasing" which means your blood sugar level is raised slowly largely due to the fiber and the nutrients. This avoids the **inflammation** that occurs in the body when you consume "fast-releasing" carbohydrates refined carbs such as: ***Sugar, white flour products, desserts, white rice*** etc. that are devoid of fiber and nutrients that help prevent inflammation and eventual weight gain. Fiber slows down the release of sugar into the blood.

Note: Potatoes are a refined carbohydrate and considered a faster-releasing food which means that the potato spikes your blood sugar level creating insulin rush and eventual weight gain. However, sweet potatoes, despite their sweetness are a slow-releasing sugar tuber.

Salt

Minimize salt. Do not add too much salt to your food when cooking or eating. Avoid very salty foods such as pork, ham, bacon, tomato juice or veggie juice (opt for low-sodium), salted nuts, bouillon, canned soups, cheese, salted crackers, snack foods, seasoned salt, soy or Worcestershire sauce, catsup, canned meats or fish, corned beef, sausage, peanut butter and foods labeled as having a high sodium content.

Get in the habit of using high-flavor ingredients, like fresh herbs, zesty spices and seasonal fruits to invigorate dishes, rather than an excess of salt.

Why Inflammation Creates Weight Gain

If you ingest refined carbohydrates, like white flour pasta for example, you will cause the body's blood sugar levels to quickly spike and just as quickly drop. It is much like throwing a ball high up in the air and watching it fall rapidly to the ground. To compensate for this spike, insulin is secreted into the bloodstream in order to lower your blood sugar.

The higher levels of insulin from refined carbs, such as with sugar, signal the body to store the excess carbohydrates as fat and to not release the fat for energy by inhibiting the action of an important enzyme known as HSL or hormone-sensitive lipase. HSL frees stored fat so it can be *burned* for energy. Cutting carbs boosts your HSL action! Insulin is the **"Fat Storage Hormone."**

Higher insulin levels also suppress Glucagon and growth hormones. *Glucagon burns fat and sugar. Growth hormone builds new muscle which is one important key for weight loss.* Muscle is metabolically active and burns calories even at rest. In other words, Glucagon and growth hormone promote fat burning! Insulin, however, is considered a storage hormone. It helps store vital nutrients in our muscle cells and unfortunately, also stores fat. ***This continual surge of excess insulin creates inflammation.***

The *consistent* use of carbohydrates such as **sugar, white flour products and all refined carbohydrates** (sugar, white wheat flour, white bread, desserts, chips, sodas, white rice, processed food), creates inflammation and gives rise to weight gain and eventual health problems such as heart disease and more.

Refined carbohydrates spell disaster in terms of promoting poor health and weight gain. Why? Because refined, processed carbohydrates have virtually no fiber and minimal nutrients and create inflammation. Vitamins, minerals and phytonutrients are also necessary to blunt the effects of fat storage.

Refined carbohydrates are essentially empty calories. While carbohydrates are a vital and necessary source of fuel for the body and the brain, if you eat too many of them, they will ultimately be stored as fat. If you want quick and lasting fat loss - reduce your refined carbohydrate intake.

Refined Carbohydrate List

- SUGAR (your #1 enemy): Sodas, candy, candy bars, fudge, jelly, desserts - you get the picture.

- High fructose corn syrup (toxic). HFCS is commonly added to many packaged foods, sodas and is a major contributor to inflammation and weight gain. Sources can include: sodas, maple syrup, honey, canned fruit pie filling, applesauce with added sugar, frozen fruit with sugar added and sweetened canned fruit. HFCS creates Leptin resistance - Leptin's ability to suppress appetite is key in fat loss.

- White flour products such as white bread, white pasta, bagels, bread, muffins, white rice and most packaged cereals. White flour in combination with sugar, adds even more of an inflammatory punch, if you will. Avoid all refined carbohydrates.

Even though bananas, raisins and dates are not refined, keep them to a minimum due to their very fast releasing sugars = inflammation.

*When reading labels, make sure you see the word **"whole"** before the grain type such as **"Whole Wheat Flour"** as opposed to 'Wheat Flour.'

Melt Fat With Fat

We need healthy fats to *burn fat!* The right types of fats will help you easily drop the pounds. Eat the wrong kinds of fat and you'll store fat! Omega-3 fats, will help you burn fat by helping your body respond more efficiently to a hormone called Leptin (*Leptin is the Greek word for thin*) and it is Leptin that signals your body (your brain) to suppress your appetite so that you will eat less and maintain or lose weight. Leptin also increases your metabolism by increasing your thyroid output. Essentially Leptin encourages your body to burn fat for energy.

"What happens when we don't eat enough good fat? Paradoxically, we become fat because we can't burn off excess fat." -Ron Rosedale

Part of optimal health and weight loss is making sure we have an adequate intake of essential fatty acids or good fats such as Omega 3 fats. It is vital to our health to consume essential fatty acids. They are called "essential" because we must obtain them from our diet as our bodies don't make them. These essential fats are critical for **weight loss**, proper brain functioning, thinning the blood to prevent heart attacks and strokes, control cholesterol and lipid levels, improve immune function and metabolism, *reduces inflammation* (very important) and maintains fluid balance in the body.

The best sources of essential fats are cold water

fish, fish oil supplements, flax seeds/oil, walnuts, Chia seeds, and Krill oil. I recommend a serving (3.5 oz.) of fatty fish such as: salmon, tuna or sardines 2 to 3 times per week for you. Supplementing with fish oil is a guarantee to ensure your omega 3 (essential fat) fats intake. Olive oil, flax oil, nuts, seeds, avocados and fatty fish are all very beneficial fats for your health as well, but fish oil is the fat you must incorporate for optimal health and weight loss. ***Remember: healthy fat in moderation helps burn fat.***

There is a special fat that I want to share with you – Coconut Oil. Coconut oil is essentially a *fat burning fat!* Coconut oil can rev-up your metabolism even more than protein. Medium-chain fatty acids (MCFA) shift the body's metabolism into a higher gear, so to speak, so that you burn more calories. This happens every time you ingest medium-chained fatty acids. Because MCFA increase the metabolic rate, they are dietary fats that can actually promote weight loss!

Unlike longer-chain fatty acids, the medium-chain fatty acids in coconut oil are tiny enough to enter your cells' mitochondria directly. This means your cells use the fat from coconut oil for energy instantly, instead of storing it for later use.

- ✓ Coconut oil is a thermogenic fat that boosts your metabolism, helping you to burn calories and lose fat.

- ✓ Coconut oil stabilizes blood sugar levels – an important key to reducing inflammation.
- ✓ Replacing other fats with coconut oil means that the rate at which your body stores fat slows down
- ✓ You will have increased energy levels and you will tend to eat less sugary and starchy foods, because you will not have the need for them.
- ✓ Coconut oil actually increases the rate at which you burn *stored fat*, even beyond the extra fat you burn simply because you exercise.

So make the switch from all of the other fats you are using to coconut oil or butter and watch your waistline shrink!

Add a healthy fat with each meal and each snack as the fat helps absorb the nutrients.

Use olive oil or coconut oil for your primary cooking fat - not butter, margarine, lard, corn oil, safflower oil or bacon fat.

Fiber and Fat Release

Fiber is vital to weight loss and optimal health. It promotes digestive health. Fiber helps produce beneficial bacteria for weight loss (beneficial bacteria also known as 'probiotics' can help burn off belly fat), optimum immune function, removes toxins, prevents certain diseases (heart disease, cancer, diabetes etc) and **Fiber keeps weight under control!**

Incorporate 8-10 grams of fiber at each meal. It's easy to do once you have the groceries in your house.

Examples of high fiber choices:

- 1 slice of sprouted whole wheat bread is an average of 4 grams of fiber per slice. Top with a slice of low-fat cheese, add a glass of low-sodium V-8 juice = 2 grams of fiber and a piece of fruit or added salad, and there you have it!

- For breakfast, a high fiber, high protein cereal such as a whole sprouted grain cereal will give you 6-8 grams of fiber per serving and top the cereal with about 10 walnut halves and quarter cup of blueberries.

- Dinner can include a whole wheat low-carb tortilla that averages10 grams of fiber filled with one serving of salmon, topped with a couple slices of avocado and salsa.

Water and Fat Loss

Water is your fat loss friend and just like a good friend, it is good for you.

It is *extremely* important to have an adequate water intake each day. Drink half your body weight in ounces of water daily. For example, if you weigh 120 pounds you need to drink a minimum of 60 ounces.

Most people are walking around mildly dehydrated suffering symptoms and do not even realize it. They are feeling *hunger*, fatigue, joint pain, headaches, lethargy, back pain and much more.

Water is critical for weight loss. Why? Our bodies are 75% water and our brain is 80% water. When the cells do not have adequate hydration, such as occurs with mild dehydration, our cells slow down and guess what? So does our metabolism. Adequate water intake is necessary for quick and successful weight loss.

Water takes vital nutrients to each cell in the body - to nourish our cells. Water is also a fantastic weight loss tool - not only because it creates optimal functioning cells and makes you feel fuller, but because it literally flushes the fat metabolites out of the fat cell, shrinking the cell and thus, shrinking you. Water also increases metabolism by 30% for an hour after drinking it.

Most importantly, however, water rids the body of toxins.

Many people are under the mistaken impression that drinking water causes bloating or water retention - when in fact *water prevents and alleviates it.*

A 2010 study found that drinking two glasses of water right before meals helped people lose 5 pounds more over 12 weeks than people who did not increase their water intake.

To encourage you to drink more, start the day out with water. Keep a glass of water on your nightstand and as soon as you awaken, drink up.

Bring a bottle of water with you wherever you go. Keep a glass or bottle of water on your desk at work to drink and refill when empty.

If needed, use a reminder alarm on your phone or calendar or put a sticky note on your computer

Give water more flavor by adding fresh orange, lemon, lime or even cucumber slices, this will encourage you to drink more.

If you have a craving for any type of food or feel hungry - try drinking water first. It may disappear with the water intake because the brain confuses mild dehydration with hunger.

*By the time we are thirsty, we are all ready 1-2% dehydrated.

QUICK FAT LOSS FITNESS

What if I told you that you DO NOT have to hop on a treadmill or an elliptical for what seems to be an eternity..? What if I told you that in just minutes, 3-4 times a week, would be all you needed to build real heart strength, lung power, create more energy and vigor than traditional cardio, *burn fat faster* - even while resting? You can with **High Intensity Interval Training (HIIT)**. HIIT is simply short bursts of exertion followed by rest and recovery.

Doing HIIT teaches your body to burn fat and build muscle, it greatly increases your lung capacity, turns your body into a fat burning machine with strong muscles and youthful features.

Remember, it's all about fat loss - right?

HIIT really boils down to engaging all three of your muscle fibers: Fast-twitch, slow-twitch and super-fast-twitch muscle fibers to create *amazing* fitness, health and weight loss, *especially the fast twitch muscles* that traditional long slower cardio doesn't touch…and your time investment to reap the benefits? Minimal.

Remember, it's about increasing the speed of your fat loss, right?

This is why, even though you are grueling away on the treadmill for hours a week, you're not seeing results! Why? Because the biggest changes occur *after* not during the exercise. Your metabolism is affected for several days afterward. So just using the other half of your muscle fibers, your fast-twitch muscles, and you see excellent results!

When you do traditional long cardio, you only work the slow-twitch muscles, but not the fast and super-fast twitch muscles which are the ones that release Human Growth Hormone. **Human Growth Hormone** is *key* for optimal fitness and more. HIIT increases fat loss by boosting human growth hormone production and is often referred to as "the fitness hormone." People with the highest levels of HGH are generally the healthiest, leanest and fittest. And guess what? You can have this in only minutes 3-4 times a week!

Here are a few examples of HIIT workouts you might like to try:

- **The *'P.A.C.E.'* workout in total is 12 minutes, 3-4 times a week. This workout starts out with low intensity for four minutes with complete rest until recovered after each set. All sets (4 minutes, 3 minutes, 2 minutes, 1 minute) become shorter, yet more intense. Frequency is 3-4 times weekly.**

- **The *'Peak Fitness'* workout is a 30 second workout with 90 seconds low intensity recovery. Repeat 8 times. Frequency is 3-4 times weekly.**

- *'Tabata'* is a 20 seconds workout with 10 seconds rest. Repeat 8 times. Frequency is 2- 4 times weekly.

- *'The Little Method'* is a high intensity 60 second workout with 75 seconds of low intensity recovery. Repeat 12 times. Frequency is 3 times weekly.

Note:

HIIT can be done on a treadmill and/or an elliptical trainer. Just go at it the same way as you would when sprinting. In fact, it's a great way for indoor training. Just make sure to use your whole body, including swinging your arms, when doing this for maximum return. You would sprint for a given amount of time, followed by a rest period or a walk.

Other ways to do indoor HIIT would be doing exercises like burpees, squat thrusts, jumping jacks, rope skipping or jumping lunges. All will work your whole body when done correctly. If you have knee problems, then do the squat thrusts. Always keep proper form when performing any exercise. This will help prevent injury.

If you're training outside, then you can sprint, bicycle, swim, hill runs (if you have one near) and run stairs – all using the various methods of HIIT.

Let me add one final exercise routine that simulates HIIT. It's called circuit training. You would basically do 5-10 different exercises at about 10-15 repetitions. There is no rest between exercises and only about a 1 minute rest period between circuits. And then you would repeat the circuits until you reach your time limit. That could be anywhere from 10-20 minutes.

Keeping proper form is important in any type of exercise routine. That includes HIIT and circuits. The alignment of musculoskeletal system will help to ensure that injuries are minimized. Do HIIT as fast as possible and only as fast as your form remains good.

Before you begin any exercise routine and especially ones that are higher intensity, make sure to get a check-up from your physician.

A Basic 5 Exercise Circuit

1. Push-ups

2. Squats

3. Pull-ups or bodyweight rows (this can be substituted for elastic band standing rows)

4. Squat thrusts

5. Reverse crunches

Push-ups: When engaged in doing push-ups, make sure to keep your abs and glutes tight. If you can't do a complete push-up, then elevate your body until you can to them. I would suggest using the top of a table to 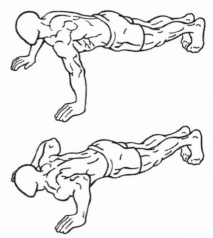 plant your hands as you keep your feet on the ground. You can also use a wall.

The reason you want to do push-ups this instead of many trainers telling you to put your knees on the ground is that it helps to develop a strong core. You will get a double benefit by keeping your whole body inline, almost like being in a plank.

Squats:
Many people have knee problem when doing squats and simply stop. Squats are one of the exercises 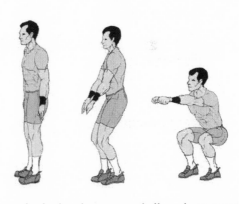 that work your whole body, especially when you

add resistance to it. For this exercise, concentrate on using your own bodyweight. If you are overweight, then you won't need any added resistance.

When doing squats, make sure your feet are shoulder width apart and feet pointed straight ahead. As you start to squat down, your knees should not go past the ends of your toes. Adjust your squat so that you won't put the kind of stress on it that most people do.

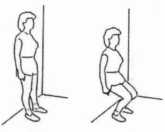

You can also use a ball against the wall. Simply position yourself with your back against the ball and squat down. You can move your feet out so that your knees keep from extending past your toes. This will work your thighs more intensely. Going slower or faster will increase the intensity in different ways. Experiment for yourself.

Adding jumps to your squats creates explosive strength and brings in more muscle fibers. Again, experiment to see what works for you. Another good way to build your legs when doing squats is by doing them statically. This means to keep in one position. By putting your back against a wall and going down into a nearly 90 degree position or higher, your legs will build strength. This is good when you may have bad balance, want to work on one leg or have an additional challenge.

Lunges: These work the legs along with squats.

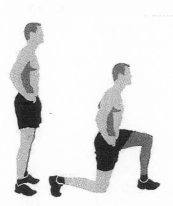

You can do them in place or walking. There are many different variations. The basic is stepping forward as you squat down. The deeper you go, the more muscles you will engage. Another benefit of deep lunges is that you will help stretch your muscles and tendons. Doing deep lunges are a form of dynamic stretching and can be done at the beginning of a workout.

Pull-ups:
These are done with your palm-grips facing outward. Chin-ups are done with

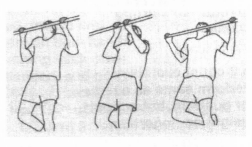

your palm-grips facing inward. When doing a

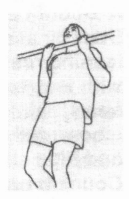

pull-up or chin-up, make sure to extend nearly all the way, just don't lock your elbows. When you pull yourself up, your chin should extend to just over the bar. Since the average man can only do about 1 pull-up, get someone to assist you. Or use a chair to stand on and for assistance.

If you are very weak, I would suggest holding yourself at the top and letting gravity bring you back down. Get help to push yourself to the top. This way you will start to build strength in your arms, shoulders and back. Eventually, you will be able to do 10 or more pull-ups without assistance. It will take time to get there.

Bodyweight (Inverted) Rows: These are done using only your bodyweight. You can use suspension straps (such as the TRX system) or hold onto a barbell (inverted). See the pic below on how it's done.

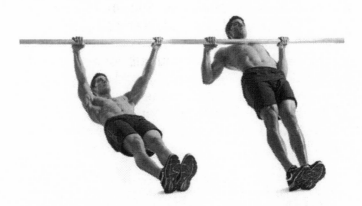

Elastic Band Rows: These are done with any type of elastic band. The goal is to make sure to pull the full length until your shoulder blades feel like they are coming together. Any style of rowing needs to ensure this happens. The benefit is that your back will get stronger and your posture will be much better.

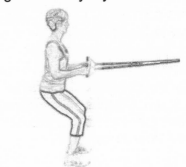

Squat Thrusts: You would start in the standing position and then go down into a squat. Put your hands on the ground in front of you for support and then throw your legs behind you into a push-up position. Next, bring your legs back into a squat and then stand up. Repeat. This is a great exercise as it works the whole body.

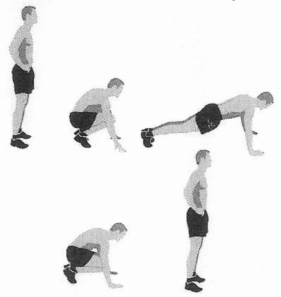

A modification of the squat thrust is called the "burpee." In essence, you'd do the same thing except you'd add a jump into the air at the end. It's more intense and really works your legs. It's also a form of plyometrics (explosive strength training).

Reverse Crunches: While many fitness advocates still teach regular crunches, they are not effective and can be damaging. Instead, do reverse crunches. They put 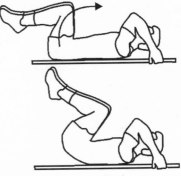 less strain on the lower back and work the abdominal muscles much better. I would do them along with the plank.

Front Plank: This is an excellent core developer and stabilizer. Make sure to tighten your abs and glutes when doing this. Hold this

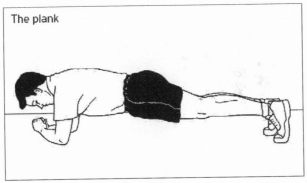

The plank

position as long as possible. I would suggest doing this as a primary core exercise.

Exercise routines

The following exercise routines suggest that you are already at a decent level of fitness.   If you are starting out, I would suggest that you engage in a 10,000 step walking exercise program. This will help get you back into shape. From there you can start out at the first circuit listed and only do one circuit.

Circuit Routine #1

Do 15 minutes of 15 each push-ups, squats, standing elastic band rows, squat thrusts and reverse crunches. Rest 30-60 seconds between circuits and repeat until you reach 15 minutes.

Circuit Routine #2:

Do 3 circuits of 20: squats, push-ups, bodyweight or standing elastic band rows, lunges, front planks (hold for 1 minute). Rest 60 seconds and repeat for 2 more circuits.

Circuit Routine #3:

Do 2-5 circuits of 15 reps: Push-ups, squats, pull-ups or rows, table-top push-ups, lunges, reverse crunches, squat thrusts, and a one minute plank. Repeat after a one minute rest.

High Intensity Interval Training (HIIT)
As previously stated, there are many variations

of HIIT. You can do them circuit style or even pick one exercise. The less rest between exercises, the more fat-burning benefit you will get. Your metabolism rate will remain much higher over the next 12-24 hours.

If you live near a track, you can do a variation where you would sprint the straight-aways and walk the curves. This will get your heart pumping in no time. I would test it out at one lap around the track to see where you are at. That means sprinting twice and walking twice. You can increase the one lap with a jog after the sprint. Then go two laps. Eventually you will be doing up to 8 laps.

You can HIIT timed too. Tabata is done this way and so are most versions of HIIT. Even in front of your TV set in your living room you can do HIIT. For example, using squat thrust or burpees, do as many as you can in 30 seconds (with proper form) and rest 1 minute, is a great HIIT workout.

Indoor HIIT

HIIT #1: Jumping lunges for one minute and rest one minute. Repeat for up to 6 total rounds.

HIIT #2: Squat thrusts for 30 seconds, rest one minute. Repeat for up to 8 total rounds.

HIIT #3: Burpees for 20 seconds, rest 30 seconds. Repeat for up to 8 total rounds.

Outdoor HIIT

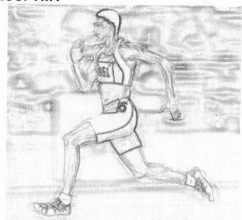

HIIT #4: Sprint for 50 meters or yards, walk back to starting position. Repeat for up a total of 8 rounds.

HIIT #5: Sprint for 50 meter or yards, do 10 push-ups, walk back to starting point and repeat for up to 8 rounds.

HIIT #6: Hit the pool with HIIT. Swim sprint 50 meters, rest for 30 seconds and repeat for up to 8 laps. For added intensity do 10 pushups after each lap.

Fun Training that Burns Fat Fast

There's no reason why you can't have fun and burn off fat fast. Have you ever watched children play? They will engage in all kinds of activities. At least they did years ago. You may even remember doing activities like bear crawls and crab walks. Playing like that will help increase your metabolic rate, especially if you do it like a kid.

Just like in HIIT, the start and stop and start again that kids will do is the same kind of action. Go at it fast and furious and then rest for about a minute. Do it again.

Fun Activity #1: Bunny Hop for 25 meters/yards and bear crawl back. Repeat for 3-4 times.

Fun Activity #2: Race to a tree for about 50 meters away, rest and then race back. Find friend or kid to challenge. Do this a total of 4 times.

Fun Activity #3: Bear Crawl 25 meters/yards, crab walk back to the start. Do as many as you can after resting for one minute.

Top Weight Loss Supplements

The following nutrients work to enhance the loss of body fat, preserve muscle mass and regulate levels of blood sugar and insulin that result in reducing cellular inflammation -- key attributes of a healthy, young body.

1. **Fish Oil.**

Fish oil is a superior supplement that will help promote weight loss by reducing inflammation in your body by decreasing insulin levels. *Fish oil supplements reduce inflammation and will help to stop the physical effects of carbohydrate consumption such as blood sugar swings allowing for weight loss and optimal health.*

DOSAGE RECOMMENDATION: 3,000 mg. per day of fish oil.

2. **Glutamine**

Glutamine plays an important role in keeping the muscles functioning properly and helps reduce muscle deterioration. Remember, muscle is metabolically active where fat just sits there and this equals calorie burn. Muscle burns calories even at rest. Glutamine drives muscle-building nitrogen into the muscle cell where it is synthesized for growth. Glutamine is also converted into glucose when the body needs more energy. When the body is in a highly inflammatory state, it breaks down our muscle tissue to get the extra glutamine needed, resulting in muscle loss.

DOSAGE RECOMMENDATION: 2,000 mg. daily

3. **Acetyl L-Carnitine**

Acetyl L-Carnitine is one of the most important nutrients for weight loss. Acetyl L-Carnitine leads to increased fat burning and helps increase your metabolism while preserving your muscle mass. Acetyl L-Carnitine is excellent for eliminating cravings and increasing the amount of energy you have to exercise. In order for Acetyl L-Carnitine to be effective, we must have adequate essential fatty acids, such as omega 3's (fish oil, walnuts, and cold water fish, etc.) in our diet.

Dosage Recommendation: 500 mg. daily.

4. **Vitamin D3**

Vitamin D3, in conjunction with calcium, helps to properly assimilate food and regulate normal blood sugar levels. When there is a lack of calcium, oftentimes due to a vitamin D deficiency, the body increases production of synthase, a fatty acid enzyme that coverts calories into fat. This explains the correlation between low levels of vitamin D, weight gain and obesity.

Dosage Recommendation: 3,000 IUs daily.

5. **Coenzyme Q10 or CoQ10**

Coenzyme Q10, also called ubiquinone, is a powerful antioxidant/anti-inflammatory that boosts metabolism and thus assisting with weight gain and obesity. It assists in energy production within the mitochondria. Because CoQ10 stokes our metabolism, it gives us increased energy and a greater ability to lose body fat.

Dosage Recommendation: 150 mg. daily

6. **Chromium Picolinate**

Because Chromium is an essential nutrient for normal sugar and fat metabolism, it is critical in our effort to control and reduce excess body fat. Chromium supplementation effectively lowers blood sugar and insulin levels, thus playing a key role in regulating appetite, reducing sugar cravings, and lowering body fat. Chromium Picolinate is highly effective in reducing sugar cravings!

Dosage Recommendation: 200 mcg. daily

7. **Maitake Mushroom Extract**

Maitake Mushroom extract enhances insulin sensitivity for controlling blood sugar levels even without lowering our caloric intake and increasing exercise. Maitake mushroom extract is also a highly effective immune booster.

Recommended Dosage: 100 mg. daily

8. **Green Tea Extract**

Green tea contains polyphenols that reduce inflammation and create thermogenesis (the metabolism is raised and fat cells are then utilized as energy, boosting the metabolic rate).

Recommended Dosage: 500 mg. Daily

9. **R-Lipoic Acid**

R-Lipoic Acid, often referred to as 'the universal antioxidant," is a potent anti-inflammatory and antioxidant. It works by helping to boost energy use by the mitochondria within the cells and promotes the metabolism of carbohydrates and sugar.

Recommended Dosage: 300 mg. daily

Think of supplements as a part of your multi-pronged approach to fat loss. Your goal is to reduce and prevent inflammation in order to lose weight and keep it off. Each of these supplements will reduce and prevent inflammation, along with helping to speed up the weight loss process in a healthy manner.

I highly recommend adding a multivitamin mineral to further reduce inflammation. Not all of us get the required nutrients from our diet for various reasons such as depleted nutrients in the soil, pesticide use, long storage life and more.

A superior resource for nutritional information regarding supplements and nutrition is the Life Extension Foundation (see Appendix A) that will be highly useful to you in your quest for weight loss, optimal health and fitness.

10. Green Coffee Bean Extract

Chlorogenic Acid in Pure Green Coffee Bean Extract has been shown to promote the liver to burn fat, increase metabolism, and inhibit fat absorption and the release of glucose into the blood after eating. Chlorogenic Acid is a natural phytochemical that is highly concentrated in Pure Green Coffee Bean Extract.

DOSAGE RECOMMENDATIONS: 400 mg. twice daily

'At A Glance' What to Eat

Here are examples of foods you can eat. Remember that there are many more healthy food choices.

Protein

Chicken Breast

Turkey Breast

Lean Ground Turkey

Salmon

Tuna

Lobster

Shrimp

Top Round Steak

Lean Ground Beef

Buffalo

Bison

Lean Ham

Eggs

Low-Fat Cottage Cheese

Fat Free Yogurt

Fat Free Milk

Wild Game Meat

Turkey Bacon

Complex Carbohydrates

Quinoa

Sweet Potato

Squash

Pumpkin

Brown Rice

Wild Rice

Beans (Black, Kidney, Red, Navy etc.)

Sprouted Whole Wheat Couscous

Kashi

Bulgur

Oatmeal

Barley

Sprouted Whole Wheat Pasta

Sprouted Whole Wheat Pita Bread

Sprouted Whole Wheat Tortillas

Low to No Sugar High Fiber Cereal

All Sprouted Whole Grains

Vegetables

All Vegetables.

Fruits

Blackberries

Raspberries

Blueberries

Strawberries

Apples

Kiwis

Lemons

Limes

Oranges

Tangerines

Grapefruit

Peaches

Plums

Pears

Plant Proteins

Quinoa

Nuts

Seeds

Legumes

Tofu

Tempeh

Edamame

Seitan

Beans

Texturized Vegetable Protein

Veggie Burgers

Healthy Fats

Avocado

Real Butter

Eggs

Seeds

Nuts

Cold Water Fish

Natural Peanut Butter

Olives

Olive Oil

Flax Oil

Krill Oil

Coconut Oil

Chia Seeds

'At A Glance' What Not To Eat

Protein

Bacon

Deep-Fried Meats - Fried Chicken, Chicken Fingers, Fish Sticks, Buffalo Wings etc.

Meats sautéed or cooked in fatty sauces or excessive amounts of oil.

Fatty Cuts of Meat

Hot Dogs

Simple Carbohydrates

Sugar

White Flour

High-Fructose Corn Syrup

Cookies

Cake

White Bread

White Rice

Crackers

Candy

French Fries

Chips

Doughnuts

Sodas

Diet Sodas

Unhealthy Fats

Fake Butter

Lard

Shortening

Full-Fat Mayonnaise

Cream Based Sauces

Full-Fat Dairy Products

Saturated Fats (are fine in moderation)

Trans Fats

Quick Tips to Fat Loss Success

"You will never change your life until you change something you do daily." *~Mike Murdock*

"Where you start is not as important as where you finish." *~Zig Ziglar*

- Eat breakfast every day! People who eat breakfast lose weight and maintain that weight loss compared to those who do not eat breakfast.

- Eat to lose weight!

- Don't skip meals! This is your quick ticket to weight gain.

- Avoid sugar. Sugar causes the release of insulin and insulin is your fat storage hormone. Sugar creates inflammation and inflammation creates weight gain.

- Avoid refined carbohydrates such as sugar, white flour, and white rice. Remember what insulin can do?

- Drink 2 glasses of water before each meal. Studies show this to be a highly effective weight loss technique.

- Eat a variety of foods. Each food has different nutrients that help prevent inflammation.

- Watch the size of your portions! For example, a whole thumb is the size of one tablespoon; the tip of your thumb to the middle joint is 1 teaspoon; your fist is about 1 cup; a 3 oz. serving of meat is about the size and thickness of your palm.

- Post a pic of whatever motivates you to stick to your goal (it works, science shows). Consider a pic of you looking healthier and leaner, someone you view as a role model in health and fitness, an upcoming event such as a wedding. Hang the picture on your fridge, put in on your phone or on your computer.

- Sleep. You need your shut-eye to avoid packing on the pounds. Aim for a minimum of 7 hours a night.

- Focus on inches lost not pounds lost.

- Read Labels Routinely

- Schedule Your Exercise and Honor It As You Would a Doctor Appointment.

- Move your body every day! High Intensity Interval Training (HIIT) is your very best weight loss friend. The best part? You don't have to do the traditional cardio for hours a week and you will burn even more fat..just minutes a day, a few times a week.

- Strength train. Muscle burns calories even at rest and is highly effective for weight loss.

- Add Whey protein to your morning meal to boost metabolism. Whey protein is one of the best ways to boost that metabolism and it makes for an easy breakfast if made into a shake or smoothie.

- Take your supplements. Supplements are meant to 'supplement' not to be confused with a magic bullet. Look at supplements as part of your overall weight loss strategy along with exercise, and smart fat loss eating.

- Use Small Plates. Studies overwhelming show we eat much less on a smaller plate. Look for a 9 inch plate to help you drop the weight.

- Use the 'Plate Method' for weight loss success. Half your plate will be veggies, 1/4 will be your lean protein and 1/4 will be your complex carbohydrates.

- Plan and prepare. Planning what you will eat and preparing some of your food in advance will make it much easier for you to create success.

- If a craving hits, commit to the '5 Minute Rule' before you eat it. Waiting five minutes will allow you to distract yourself by making a phone call, play with your children, take a car ride or take a walk. Distracting yourself works like a charm because the brain then engages in another activity. Oh and by the way, don't stare at the clock.

- Stop beating yourself up - perfection is impossible.

- When motivation wanes always go back to your 'WHY' - why you wanted weight loss in the first place - go back to the feeling part of it.

- Kick excuses to the curb.

Weight Loss Tips #2

- Make sure to set your goals! People who track their goals are the ones most likely to realize them.
- Eating 1/4 cup of walnuts daily can speed the breakdown of belly fat by 62%.
- Add whey protein to your diet every day to boost your metabolism.
- Sign up for a walk or run race for motivation and fun
- Add Capsaicin, which gives chile peppers their fire..can also fire-up your fat burn by cranking up your metabolism
- Use ground cinnamon to stabilize your blood sugar and reduce the insulin response.
- If a drink has added sugar in it, consider it *liquid fat*.
- Beware of foods with phrases such as "natural," "fat-free," "diet," or "smart choice" They tend to be buzz words and not healthy!
- Stay away from processed foods with many ingredients. Choose whole foods with one ingredient: an apple, orange, salmon, nuts..you get the picture.
- Protein at breakfast is crucial for effective fat loss. Eggs, Greek yogurt, peanut

butter etc. lead to feelings of fullness that last all day long.

- The more muscle you have the hotter your fat burn. If you activate your muscles through exercise, your fat burn lasts for up to 24 hours.

- Lightly spray or brush on the oil when grilling with pastry brush.

- Eat regular meals and avoid grazing as this contributes to weight gain.

- Try flavored coffee such as chocolate raspberry, hazelnut or vanilla for a delicious treat that is low in calories.

- Become a label detective. Read labels to help you understand their portion sizes and what you are putting into your body.

- Blueberries contain inflammation reducing anthocyanins that help prevent increased fat storage.

- Cutting out the white flour foods such as breads, pastas and pastries can jump start your fat burn' to 'Cutting out the white flour foods such as breads, pasta and pastries will jump start your fat burn.

- Eliminate all packaged foods.

- Slow down your eating. Fast eating leads straight to fat gain because there isn't adequate time for the brain to receive the message you have had enough food.

- When dining out ask the waiter for a to-go box early in the meal and eat only half your meal, then take the other half home for another meal.
- Cut a large amount of calories by ordering a skim cappuccino or flavored coffee instead of dessert.
- Stand whenever possible. Standing burns 30% more calories than sitting.
- Get rid of your "Fat Clothes." This will force you to focus and move forward.
- Learn to love soup. Soup is high in water content and has a filling effect to keep overeating and wrong food choices at bay.
- Quit mindless snacking. Take the portion with you – not the bag or box.
- Make the switch from milk to almond milk – almond milk has lowered natural sugars.
- Grab a partner. Use the buddy system to keep you accountable, focused and motivated.
- Brush your teeth after every meal. If your teeth are sparkling clean you'll be less tempted to indulge.
- Have protein and a carb after each workout – amazing results!

- Begin to move your body more in your everyday life.
- If you are short on workout time, squeeze in a workout early in the morning before the day gets started and soon it will be routine.
- Visualizing the body you want will help keep you focused and as a result, you will make those important fat-burning choices.
- Don't compare yourself to others. You are an inherently beautiful and worthwhile person who is also on a journey. Stay focused and it is yours.

YOUR FAT LOSS GOALS

"You cannot expect to achieve new goals or move beyond your present circumstances unless you change." *~Les Brown*

"Your goals, minus your doubts, equal your reality." *~Ralph Marston*

Your goals are to:

- Eat frequently throughout the day.

- Fill your grocery cart up with quality lean proteins, complex carbohydrates, fruits and veggies

- Make protein and veggies the focus of your plate.

- Integrate the *"Healthy Focus"* items on the Nutrition Fast Trac™ every day.

- Drink half your body weight in water each day.

- Take your supplements daily.

- Engage in High Intensity Interval Training (HIIT) 3-4 times a week.

- Strength training 2-3 times a week.

These weight loss goals are your core focus each day!

By implementing the above goals, you will accomplish not only rapid weight loss, but life-long optimal health as well.

"Your decisions, not the conditions of your lives, determine your destiny"
~Anthony Robbins

Appendix A: Nutrition Fast Trac™ To Weight Loss Success

Use the Nutrition Fast Trac™ for 4 weeks. Focus on these areas as designated by week.

Week 1: Water
Week 2: Portion Control
Week 3: Minimize Sugar
Week 4: Fruits & Veggies

	PROTEIN	COMPLEX CARBOHYDRATE	FRUIT/VEGGIE	HEALTHY FAT	GLASSES OF WATER
SUNDAY					
Breakfast					
Snack					
Lunch					
Snack					
Dinner					
MONDAY					
Breakfast					
Snack					
Lunch					
Snack					
Dinner					

TUESDAY					
Breakfast					
Snack					
Lunch					
Snack					
Dinner					
WEDNESDAY					
Breakfast					
Snack					
Lunch					
Snack					
Dinner					
THURSDAY					
Breakfast					
Snack					
Lunch					
Snack					
Dinner					

FRIDAY					
Breakfast					
Snack					
Lunch					
Snack					
Dinner					
SATURDAY					
Breakfast					
Snack					
Lunch					
Snack					
Dinner					

Appendix B: Sample Weekly Meal Plan

Monday - Breakfast

Spanish Eggs. Scramble 3 egg whites and 1 egg yolk in 1 tsp. olive oil. Top with salsa. 1 slice of toasted sprouted whole wheat bread. Glass of low-sodium veggie juice.

Monday - Snack

1 cup mixed berries with 1/4 cup pecans.

Monday - Lunch

Tomato and Mozzarella Salad. Sliced tomatoes, 2 thin slices of Mozzarella, red onion and an 1/8 cup of pine nuts. Drizzle with Olive oil and Balsamic vinegar. 1 serving whole grain crackers.

Monday - Snack

3 Slices Avocado with one string cheese.

Monday - Dinner

Open-Faced Roast Beef Sandwich. One slice sprouted whole wheat bread with 2 tbsp. pesto. 4 oz. deli roast beef. Spinach salad tossed with olive oil/vinegar.

Tuesday - Breakfast

Scrambled Egg Sandwich. Scramble 3 egg whites and 1 egg yolk. 1 toasted sprouted whole grain English muffin. Dijon mustard. Top with 1 oz. reduced-fat Monterey Jack cheese and 1/4 cup avocado. Veggie juice.

Tuesday - Snack

1 apple and 2 tbsp peanut butter

Tuesday - Lunch

Seafood Salad. Combine 4 oz. chunk light tuna mixed, 2 tbsp. grated reduced-fat cheddar with 1/2 cup chilled whole wheat pasta spirals. Toss with 1 tsp olive oil and balsamic vinegar, 5 sliced black olives and diced green pepper.

Tuesday - Snack

Carrots and celery with 3 tbsp Hummus dip.

Tuesday - Dinner

Tex-Mex Burger. Stuff low-carb tortilla with 1 black bean veggie burger, 1 slice reduced-fat cheddar cheese, 3 tbsp guacamole and red onion. 1 spinach salad with veggies.

Wednesday - Breakfast

Scrambled Breakfast Tacos. Scramble 3 egg whites and 1 egg yolk, fill low-carb tortilla with egg mixture and top with 2 tbsp. guacamole.

Wednesday - Snack

Handful of almonds (about 15) and an apple

Wednesday - Lunch

Tuna Pita. 4 oz. chunk light tuna combined with 2 tbsp. of Tahini past, parsley. Stuff into a whole wheat pita. Baby carrots.

Wednesday - Snack

1 cup cottage cheese and veggie juice.

Wednesday - Dinner

Grilled flank Steak 4 oz., with grilled onions, mixed green salad, olive oil, edamame beans

Thursday - Breakfast

Cheddar Melt. Top sprouted whole wheat English muffin with 2 slices reduced fat cheddar cheese. Broil. 1/2 cup melon balls.

Thursday - Snack

6 oz. fat-free plain yogurt mixed with mashed fresh raspberries and 1/8 tsp flax oil, cinnamon.

Thursday - Lunch

4 oz. grilled tuna fillet with 1/4 cup brown rice. Raw mixed veggie sticks and 2 tbs. humsus. Veggie juice.

Thursday - Snack

Hard-boiled egg. Handful of grapes.

Thursday - Dinner

Grilled or baked chicken breast. Steamed spinach with onions and mushrooms, 1/2 cup quinoa, sliced tomatoes drizzled with olive oil.

Friday - Breakfast

Lori's Luscious Smoothie. 1 scoop whey protein powder (chocolate/vanilla), half banana, handful blueberries, 1/4 tsp. cinnamon, 8 oz. no-sugar almond milk. Blend.

Friday - Snack

Oatmeal with 1/2 scoop whey protein powder and almond milk.

Friday - Lunch

Open-faced Tuna Sandwich. Water-packed canned tuna mixed with yogurt cheese, chopped celery, 1/4 cup diced avocado on top of sprouted whole grain bread. Apple.

Friday - Snack

1 handful almonds; 1 pear.

Friday - Dinner

Roasted turkey breast; steamed broccoli, brown rice.

Saturday - Breakfast

3 egg whites, 1 egg yolk scrambled with 1/4 cup reduced-fat cheddar; 1/2 sprouted grain English muffin.

Saturday - Snack

5 slices turkey with 1 peach

Saturday - Lunch

Mixed green salad. Mixed greens, chickpeas, black beans, tomatoes, celery, carrots, slivered almonds, cucumbers drizzled with olive oil.

Saturday - Snack

½ cup of blueberries; 1 handful almonds.

Saturday - Dinner

Mixed Vegan Meal. Sprouted whole wheat couscous, toasted pine nuts, grilled tempeh, steamed asparagus.

Sunday - Breakfast

Southwestern Burrito. 3 egg whites, 1 egg scrambled with black beans, avocado, tomatoes added to a sprouted whole grain wrap.

Sunday - Snack

2 tbsp. peanut butter on half sprouted English muffin.

Sunday - Lunch

Salmon Stuffed Tomatoes. 6 oz. tuna mixed with chopped tomatoes; celery; 1/4 cup Greek yogurt; 1 tbsp. olive oil and stuffed into tomatoes.

Sunday - Snack

1 handful of walnuts; apple

Sunday - Lunch

English Muffin Pizza. 1/2 sprouted whole grain English muffin, tomato sauce, 2 tbsp. reduced-fat cheddar cheese, 2 tbsp. fat free cottage cheese, cut-up veggies. Mixed baby greens salad drizzled with olive oil.

Sunday - Snack

Hummus Snack Wrap. Spread 2 tbsp. hummus, add fat-free feta cheese, roasted red peppers onto a low-carb wrap.

Sunday - Dinner

Turkey Chili. Simmer 1 lb. ground turkey, onion, celery, bell pepper, garlic, in 2 tbsp. olive oil, add 3 cans beans, 2 cans diced tomatoes, 1 qt chicken broth, chili powder.

FIRE-UP YOUR FAT BURN! RECIPES

SOUTHWESTERN OMELETTE

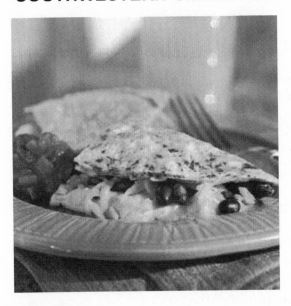

Ingredients
- 2 tablespoons chopped fresh cilantro
- 1/4 teaspoon salt
- 4 large egg whites
- 1 large egg
- 1/2 cup canned black beans, rinsed and drained
- 1/4 cup chopped green onions

- 1/4 cup (1 ounce) reduced-fat shredded cheddar cheese
- 1/4 cup salsa
- Cooking spray

Directions

1.   Combine first 4 ingredients in a medium bowl, stirring with a whisk. Combine beans, onions, cheese, and salsa in a medium bowl.

2.   Heat a medium nonstick skillet coated with cooking spray over medium heat. Pour egg mixture into pan; let egg mixture set slightly. Tilt pan and carefully lift edges of omelet with a spatula; allow uncooked portion to flow underneath cooked portion. Cook 3 minutes; flip omelet. Spoon bean mixture onto half of omelet. Carefully loosen omelet with a spatula; fold in half. Cook 1 minute or until cheese melts. Slide omelet onto a plate; cut in half.

Nutrition Information

Amount per serving
- Calories: 181
- Calories from fat: 27%
- Fat: 5.5g
- Saturated fat: 2.3g
- Monounsaturated fat: 1g
- Polyunsaturated fat: 0.8g
- Protein: 20.2g

- Carbohydrate: 13.8g
- Fiber: 6g
- Cholesterol: 116mg
- Iron: 2.1mg
- Sodium: 522mg
- Calcium: 184mg

TURKEY BLACK BEAN SUN-DRIED TOMATO AND AVOCADO WRAP

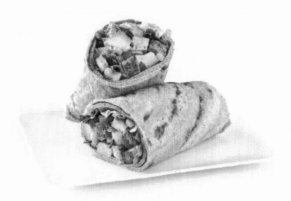

Ingredients

- 1 cup canned black beans rinsed
- 1/2 cup chopped fresh tomato
- 1/4 cup chopped soft sun-dried tomatoes
- 1 Tablespoon olive oil
- 1 tablespoon red-wine vinegar or cider vinegar
- 8 thin slices low-sodium deli turkey (about 8 ounces)
- 4 8-inch low carb wraps or low- carb whole-wheat tortillas
- 2 cups chopped romaine lettuce
- 2 slices of avocado

Directions

1. Combine black beans, tomato, sun-dried tomatoes, oil and vinegar in a medium bowl.

2. Divide deli turkey among tortillas. Top with equal portions of the black bean mixture, avocado and lettuce. Roll up. Serve the wraps cut in half, if desired.

Nutrition Information

Amount Per Serving:

- 315 calories
- 12 g fat (1 g sat , 5 g mono)
- 35 mg cholesterol
- 25 g carbohydrates
- 0 g added sugars
- 19 g protein
- 5 g fiber
- 582 mg sodium
- 325 mg potassium

Salmon Steaks with Cream Cheese

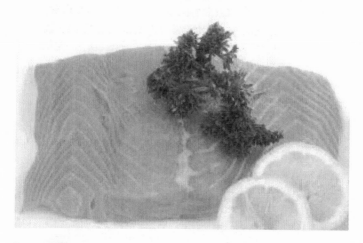

Ingredients

4 salmon steaks, 1" thick
1 T. chopped parsley
1 t. dried basil
1 T. olive oil
1/4 t. salt
4 oz. low-fat cream cheese
2 T. grated parmesan cheese
1 T. chopped green onion
2 T. lemon juice
1/4 t. pepper
4 toothpicks

Directions
Rinse steaks with cold water, pat dry. Through
the round part of the steaks make a cut to the
center, creating a pocket. Combine cheese,

parsley, basil, and green onions. Divide mixture evenly into 6 parts, form flat ovals, place one in each steak pocket, securing with a toothpick. Place steaks on oiled broiler pan. Combine olive oil, lemon juice, salt and pepper. Baste steaks with mixture. Broil 4-5 inches from heat for 4-5 minutes on each side or until flaky. Sprinkle with parmesan cheese.

Amount Per Serving

Calories	134.6
Potassium	46.5 mg
Protein	5.4 g
Total Carbohydrate	14.0 g
Cholesterol	29.0 mg
Total Fat	6.4 g
Sodium	143.4 mg
Dietary Fiber	1.1 g
Sugars	0.2 g

Thyme Coated Pork Tenderloins

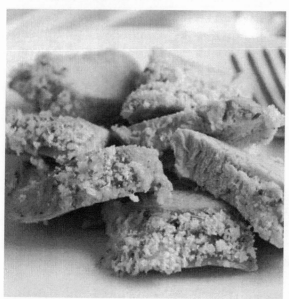

Ingredients

- 1 teaspoon dried thyme
- 1 teaspoon instant onion flakes
- 2 cups whole wheat panko (or any day old sprouted bread)
- 2 large egg whites, lightly beaten
- 1 (1-pound) pork tenderloin, trimmed
- 1/4 teaspoon salt
- 1/4 teaspoon freshly ground black pepper
- Cooking spray

Directions

1. Preheat oven to 400°.

2. Place thyme, onion, and bread in a food

processor; pulse until fine breadcrumbs measure 1/3 cup. Place breadcrumb mixture in a shallow dish. Place egg whites in a shallow dish. Sprinkle pork with salt and pepper. Dip pork in egg whites; dredge in breadcrumb mixture. Place pork on a broiler pan coated with cooking spray. Bake at 400° for 30 minutes or until a thermometer registers 155°. Let stand 5 minutes. Cut into 1/4-inch-thick slices.

Nutrition Information

Amount per serving
- Calories: 165
- Calories from fat: 22%
- Fat: 4.1g
- Saturated fat: 1.3g
- Monounsaturated fat: 1.5g
- Polyunsaturated fat: 0.3g
- Protein: 25.1g
- Carbohydrate: 5.5g
- Fiber: 0.8g
- Cholesterol: 63mg
- Iron: 1.7mg
- Sodium: 267mg
- Calcium: 17mg

Asian Flounder

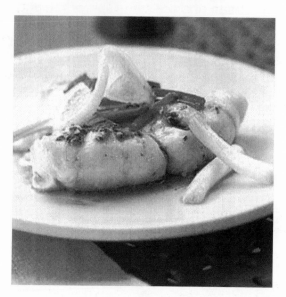

Ingredients:
- 8 green onions
- 1/4 cup minced fresh cilantro
- 1 tablespoon minced peeled fresh ginger
- 2 teaspoons dark sesame oil, divided
- 4 (6-ounce) flounder fillets, skinned
- 2 teaspoons rice vinegar
- 2 teaspoons low-sodium soy sauce
- 4 lemon slices

Directions

1. Remove green tops from onions; slice onion tops into 1-inch pieces to measure 1/4 cup; set aside. Reserve remaining onion tops for another use. Cut white portions of onions into 2-inch pieces.

2. Combine cilantro, ginger, and 1 teaspoon oil in a 9-inch pie plate. Fold each fillet in half crosswise. Arrange fish spoke like with thinnest portions pointing toward center of dish. Arrange white onion portions between each fillet. Combine 1/4 cup green onion tops, 1 teaspoon oil, vinegar, soy sauce, and salt; pour over fish. Cover with heavy-duty plastic wrap. Microwave at HIGH 4 minutes or until fish flakes easily when tested with a fork. Garnish each fillet with a lemon slice.

Nutrition Information

Amount per serving
- Calories: 188
- Calories from fat: 21%
- Fat: 4.4g
- Saturated fat: 0.8g
- Monounsaturated fat: 1.3g
- Polyunsaturated fat: 1.5g
- Protein: 32.8g
- Carbohydrate: 2.7g
- Fiber: 0.9g
- Cholesterol: 82mg

- Iron: 1.3mg
- Sodium: 299mg
- Calcium: 57mg

BON APPÉTIT!

Bonus: Motivational and Inspiring Quotes to Keep You Going

"No matter who you are, no matter what you do, you absolutely, positively do have the power to change." *~Bill Phillips*

"Within you right now is the power to do things you never dreamed possible. This power becomes available to you just as soon as you can change your beliefs." *~Dr. Maxwell Maltz*

"Act as if it were impossible to fail." *~Dorothea Brande*

One should eat to live, not live to eat. *~Cicero*

"The way to develop self-confidence is to do the thing you fear." *~William Jennings Bryan*

"You are braver than you believe, stronger than you seem, and smarter than you think." *~Christopher Robin*

"The key to change… is to let go of fear." *~Rosanne Cash*

"Life expectancy would grow by leaps and bounds if green vegetables smelled as good as bacon." *~Doug Larson*

"Courage is not the absence of fear, but rather the judgment that something else is more important than fear." *~Ambrose Redmoon*

"Act as if everything you do makes a difference. It does." *~William James*

"You are the only problem you will ever have and you are the only solution." *~Bob Proctor*

"None of us can change our yesterdays but all of us can change our tomorrows." *~Colin Powell*

"Motivation is what gets you started. Habit is what keeps you going." *~Jim Rohn*

"In order to change we must be sick and tired of being sick and tired." *~Unknown*

"Never look back unless you are planning to go that way." *~Henry David Thoreau*

"It's never too late - in fiction or in life - to revise." *~Nancy Thayer*

"Don't dwell on what went wrong. Instead, focus on what to do next. Spend your energies on moving forward toward finding the answer." *~Denis Waitley*

"Living a healthy lifestyle will only deprive you of poor health, lethargy, and fat." *~Jill Johnson*

"Take time to deliberate, but when the time for action has arrived, stop thinking and go in." *~Napoleon Bonaparte*

"Your decisions, not the conditions of your lives, determine your destiny" *~Anthony Robbins*

Resources

www.nutridiary.com
Nutridiary is a free online food and exercise diary.

Eatery.massivehealth.com
The Eatery iPhone app is the easiest way to eat healthy. Spending just a few seconds before each meal to snap a photo and rate the food, you'll get a big-picture breakdown of your habits, including your strengths, weaknesses, and the best places to start making a change.

www.platemethod.com
This site is excellent to help with weight loss in a variety of ways including the 'Plate Method.' They also have tools and products to help achieve success.

www.sparkpeople.com
This is an excellent site devoted to weight loss. It has an excellent array of weight loss tools and information.

www.calorieking.com
You can use this site to find nutrient information on most foods.

www.fitday.com
FitDay is a free online diet journal and fitness goal tracker.

www.3FatChicks.com
If you are looking for a forum, this is a great place to find support and answers.

www.lef.org
Life Extension Foundation is an excellent resource that is a global authority on nutrition, nutritional supplements, health and wellness.

www.nutrition.gov
This site will give you all you need to know about nutrition - your foundation to optimal health and weight loss.

https://www.presidentschallenge.org/
The President's Challenge assists, informs, and inspires people on their journey to be active, eat well, and get fit.

###

About Me

DR. LORI SHEMEK is known for her ability to connect with her audiences through her personal story of childhood challenges and the role inflammation played within her family that ultimately led to her passion in helping other create positive healthy change. Also known as "The Inflammation Terminator", she has made it her mission to educate the public on the toxic effects of sugar and how it creates inflammation in the body. Her expertise drew the attention of THE WOMAN'S INFORMATION NETWORK, where she has her own show on health.

Her international reputation has drawn rave revues that in 2010, The Huffington Post named Dr. Shemek one of the TOP 16 HEALTH AND FITNESS EXPERTS alongside such names as Dr. Oz. She is also a health expert for the ABC show, GOOD MORNING TEXAS. She is a leading authority on inflammation and its role in weight loss, preventing disease and optimizing health.

Dr. Shemek holds a Doctorate in Psychology; she is a Certified Nutritional Consultant and a Certified Life Coach.

She has appeared on numerous radio talk shows (highly sought after) as well as TV; has authored numerous articles and is actively doing speaking engagements for organizations, large and small.

Connect with me:

Twitter: **www.twitter.com/LoriShemek**

Facebook:
www.facebook.com/DrLoriShemek

My Blog: **LoriShemek.net**

My Website: **www.dlshealthworks.com**

41646383R00067

Made in the USA
Lexington, KY
21 May 2015